The Focused Rebellion:
A Man's Guide to Overcoming ADHD

MASTER YOUR MIND AND TRANSFORM YOUR LIFE

HENRI BEAUCHAMP

ISBN: 9798392999033

CONTENTS

CHAPTER 1: INTRODUCTION: UNDERSTANDING ADULT ADHD AND ITS IMPACT ON MEN

Welcome to "The Focused Rebellion: A Man's Guide to Overcoming ADHD," a book born out of my personal journey with Adult ADHD. As a man who has grappled with ADHD, I know firsthand the challenges and unique experiences that come with this often misunderstood condition. It was through my own need to better understand and live with ADHD that I discovered the strategies and insights that I now want to share with you.

If you're a man living with ADHD or suspect that you might be, this book is your roadmap to navigating the chaos, embracing your unique gifts, and turning ADHD into a source of strength.

ADHD, or Attention Deficit Hyperactivity Disorder, is a neurodevelopmental condition that affects millions of people worldwide. While most people think of children when they hear about ADHD, it doesn't just disappear when you grow up. In fact, it can continue to impact your life in various ways as an adult.

This book is tailored specifically for men with ADHD, as we face a unique set of challenges and experiences that differ from women and children. In the pages that follow, we will dive deep into the world of Adult ADHD in men, exploring its symptoms, the diagnostic process, and the common misconceptions surrounding the condition. We'll also discuss the personal and professional struggles that men with ADHD often face and provide strategies to help you cope and thrive in your daily life.

But understanding ADHD is only half the battle. To truly make the most of our potential, we need actionable guidance on how to harness our ADHD superpowers. That's why this book is packed with practical exercises and techniques that I've personally found helpful in managing my ADHD, and which I believe can benefit you too. From improving your focus and time management skills to building and maintaining healthy relationships, we've got you covered.

As you progress through the chapters, you'll find inspiring success stories of men who have learned to manage their ADHD and excel in various aspects of life. We'll also provide resources and support options for both you and your loved ones because no one should navigate this journey alone.

So, are you ready to join the focused rebellion and take control of your ADHD? Let's embark on this journey together, and show the world that ADHD isn't a limitation; it's a hidden superpower waiting to be unleashed.

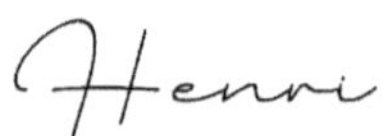

CHAPTER 2: MY JOURNEY WITH ADHD: PERSONAL INSIGHTS AND LESSONS LEARNED

Discovering My ADHD: A Life-Changing Realization

It wasn't until I turned 37 that I became aware of my ADHD, thanks to my wife's observations about my focus and inattentiveness in our relationship. Looking back, I now recognize early signs of ADHD from my childhood, such as being seemingly deaf to my mother's calls while engrossed in watching TV. At the time, my mother believed it was a hearing issue, but now I understand it was likely ADHD.

Navigating the Emotional Roller Coaster of Diagnosis

No one had ever suggested that my habits or symptoms might be due to ADHD until my wife researched and brought it up. After taking a few online tests and consulting a psychotherapist, my wife's suspicions were confirmed. Initially, I felt disappointed and even emasculated, but as I learned more about ADHD, I realized it was something I could adapt to and even leverage to my advantage.

Facing Personal and Professional Challenges with ADHD

ADHD has posed challenges in both my personal and professional life, particularly with short-term memory. I found that stress and inattention exacerbated my forgetfulness, leading to unintended consequences in my work and family life. As a husband and father, I've encountered difficulties due to my inattentiveness, from minor missteps like making too much porridge for my daughter to forgetting essentials when leaving the house. These small, thoughtless actions created unwanted stress in our lives.

Developing Coping Strategies and Techniques for Managing ADHD

One of the first steps I took was educating myself about ADHD, which ultimately inspired me to write this book. I found that resources specifically targeting men with ADHD were scarce, so I hope this book can help others like me learn and grow.

My current lifestyle doesn't always allow for consistent meditation, so I find moments throughout my day to practice mindfulness, such as when I'm soothing my daughter to sleep or feeding her. During these times, I focus on my breath or express gratitude, which helps me stay positive and resilient.

Breakthrough Moments and Realizations in My ADHD Journey
A significant breakthrough came when I started seeing a psychotherapist who
provided a safe space for me to process my thoughts and explore the root
causes of my struggles. Sharing your thoughts with a trusted friend or family
member could also help declutter your mind, benefiting your development
and mental health.

**Practical Exercises for Improving Focus, Time Management,
and Relationships**
In addition to using daily moments with my daughter to practice mindfulness,
I employ several tools to improve focus and time management. One such tool
is the Pomodoro technique, where I set a 25-minute timer to concentrate on a
single task, followed by a 5-minute break. I use my smartphone or a Google
timer for this purpose. Another tool I utilize is the Momentum Chrome
extension, which prompts me to set a daily main focus and track its
completion. These strategies help me stay attentive and mindful throughout
the day.

CHAPTER 3: EMBRACING THE SPECTRUM: ADHD IN MEN VS. WOMEN AND CHILDREN

ADHD, or Attention Deficit Hyperactivity Disorder, is a neurodevelopmental condition characterized by a range of symptoms that can impact an individual's attention, impulse control, and activity levels. While the core symptoms of ADHD are generally consistent across different age groups and genders, the way these symptoms manifest can vary significantly among men, women, and children.

In children, ADHD is often characterized by excessive restlessness, difficulty paying attention, and impulsive behavior. These symptoms can affect both boys and girls, but boys are more likely to be diagnosed with ADHD, partly because their symptoms tend to be more noticeable and disruptive.

In contrast, adult ADHD can present differently, and the distinction between men and women becomes more pronounced. Men with ADHD often exhibit externalizing symptoms such as impulsivity, hyperactivity, and difficulty with time management. These symptoms can lead to challenges in their careers, relationships, and daily functioning. Men are also more likely to exhibit aggressive or risk-taking behavior, which can further complicate their lives and create additional challenges.

On the other hand, women with ADHD are more likely to experience internalizing symptoms such as inattentiveness, disorganization, and emotional dysregulation. Their symptoms may be less obvious and can often be misattributed to anxiety or mood disorders, leading to a higher risk of underdiagnosis or misdiagnosis.

Understanding these variations in ADHD symptoms and their manifestation across different age groups and genders is crucial for accurate diagnosis, appropriate treatment, and effective management of the condition. By being aware of these differences, individuals with ADHD, their families, and healthcare professionals can better tailor their approach to address the unique challenges each person may face.

Understanding the ADHD Brain: How ADHD Manifests in Men

ADHD is a neurodevelopmental disorder characterized by difficulties with attention, impulsivity, and hyperactivity. While ADHD affects both men and women, the way it manifests can differ between the genders. For men, ADHD may present itself in the following ways:

Inattention: Men with ADHD may have trouble maintaining focus on tasks, be easily distracted, or struggle to follow through on projects.

Hyperactivity: Some men with ADHD may display physical restlessness, such as constant fidgeting, difficulty sitting still, or engaging in excessive physical activity.

Impulsivity: Men with ADHD might act without thinking, struggle with patience, or have difficulty waiting their turn in social situations.

Emotional dysregulation: Emotional sensitivity and mood swings can be more pronounced in men with ADHD, leading to challenges in interpersonal relationships and emotional well-being.

Understanding the unique ways ADHD manifests in men can help to identify symptoms, seek appropriate support, and develop tailored strategies for managing the condition.

Common ADHD Symptoms in Men: Prevalence and Manifestation

While both men and women with ADHD share the core symptoms of the disorder, some manifestations tend to be more prevalent or noticeable in men. The reasons behind these differences can be attributed to a combination of biological, social, and cultural factors. Let's take a closer look at some common ADHD symptoms that are more frequently observed in men:

Impulsivity and risk-taking behavior: Men with ADHD often exhibit higher levels of impulsivity, which can lead to a greater propensity for risk-taking behavior. This might include engaging in dangerous activities, making impulsive financial decisions, or having difficulty resisting temptations. These tendencies can result in a variety of consequences, from minor inconveniences to significant life challenges.

Hyperactivity: Although both men and women with ADHD can experience hyperactivity, it tends to be more prominent in men. This symptom can manifest as restlessness, fidgeting, or an inability to sit still for extended periods. In some cases, men with ADHD may channel their hyperactivity into excessive exercise or engaging in multiple activities at once, leading to feelings of being constantly "on the go."

Anger and aggression: Men with ADHD are more likely to display anger and aggression in response to frustration or perceived threats. This may result from difficulties in emotional regulation or impulsivity, which can make it challenging for men with ADHD to control their reactions in tense situations.

Difficulty with time management: Men with ADHD often struggle with time management and organization, leading to issues such as procrastination, missed deadlines, and frequent tardiness. These challenges can impact their professional and personal lives, creating additional stress and frustration.

Mindlessness: Men with ADHD may experience mindlessness, which refers to a lack of awareness or attentiveness to their surroundings or current tasks. This can lead to forgetfulness, difficulties in completing tasks, and a tendency to overlook important details. Over time, these challenges can contribute to feelings of inadequacy and frustration, further exacerbating the symptoms of ADHD.

It's important to note that these symptoms can vary significantly among individuals with ADHD, and not all men will experience these specific manifestations. By recognizing and understanding these common symptoms in men, healthcare professionals, individuals with ADHD, and their loved ones can develop tailored strategies and interventions to address the unique challenges they may face.

Unique Challenges Faced by Men with ADHD

Men with ADHD face a variety of unique challenges due to the interaction of their ADHD symptoms with societal expectations and their specific life circumstances. Let's explore some of these challenges:

Work and career: Men with ADHD often struggle with organization, time management, and attention to detail, which can lead to difficulties in the workplace. They may experience job dissatisfaction, frequent job changes, or underemployment as they try to find a suitable career path that accommodates their ADHD symptoms.

Relationships and family life: ADHD can impact various aspects of a man's relationships, from romantic partnerships to parenting. Men with ADHD may have difficulty with communication, emotional regulation, and maintaining consistency in their family life. This can result in strained relationships and challenges in fulfilling their roles as partners or fathers.

Masculine stereotypes: Societal expectations of men can exacerbate the challenges faced by men with ADHD. Traditional masculine roles often emphasize self-sufficiency, emotional stoicism, and problem-solving skills, which may be at odds with the realities of living with ADHD. Men with ADHD may feel shame or embarrassment about their symptoms, leading to a reluctance to seek help or disclose their condition to others.

Self-esteem and self-worth: The ongoing difficulties faced by men with ADHD can contribute to feelings of low self-esteem and self-worth. They may develop a negative self-image and feel inadequate or incompetent, which can impact their mental health and overall well-being.

Mental health: Men with ADHD are at an increased risk for developing comorbid mental health conditions, such as anxiety, depression, and substance use disorders. The unique challenges they face, combined with societal expectations and a lack of understanding about ADHD, can exacerbate these mental health issues.

To help men with ADHD overcome these unique challenges, it is essential to provide tailored support and interventions that address their specific needs. By fostering a greater understanding of the challenges faced by men with ADHD, we can help them develop effective coping strategies and improve their overall quality of life.

CHAPTER 4: DECODING ADHD: CHALLENGES AND STRENGTHS UNIQUE TO MEN

The Role of Childhood Trauma in the Development of ADHD Research has shown that traumatic experiences during childhood can increase the risk of developing ADHD in adulthood. Childhood trauma can take many forms, including physical or emotional abuse, neglect, or the experience of a family member's mental illness or substance abuse. A study by Teicher et al. (2016) found that adults with ADHD were more likely to have experienced childhood maltreatment than those without the disorder. Another study by Stevens et al. (2016) found that childhood emotional abuse was a significant predictor of adult ADHD symptoms.

Trauma can affect the developing brain and alter its structure and function, leading to changes in attention and executive function. The brain's response to trauma can result in the development of coping mechanisms that may present as ADHD symptoms in adulthood. For example, a child who experiences frequent arguments between parents may develop hyperactivity or impulsivity as a coping mechanism to deal with the stressful situation.

It's important to note that not all adults with ADHD have experienced childhood trauma, and not all individuals who experience childhood trauma develop ADHD. However, understanding the potential role of trauma in the development of ADHD can provide valuable insights into the disorder's complexities and inform tailored approaches to treatment and management.

The Challenges of ADHD in Men: Common Struggles and Areas of Difficulty
Men with ADHD face a variety of challenges in their daily lives. These challenges may include:

Time management: Difficulty organizing and prioritizing tasks, struggling with punctuality, and constantly feeling rushed or overwhelmed.

Relationships: Challenges in maintaining healthy relationships due to impulsivity, emotional dysregulation, or poor communication skills.

Work performance: Inattention and disorganization can lead to decreased productivity, missed deadlines, or conflicts with colleagues.

Self-esteem: The difficulties associated with ADHD may contribute to feelings of inadequacy, low self-esteem, or a sense of failure.

Co-existing conditions: Men with ADHD may also experience other mental health conditions, such as anxiety, depression, or substance abuse, which can compound their struggles.

Recognizing these challenges is the first step toward developing strategies to overcome them and improve overall quality of life.

Take the next step in your journey to overcome ADHD.
Download the 'Identifying Your ADHD Challenges' workbook and dive deeper into the strategies and exercises that will help you reach your goals.
https://swiy.co/adhd-challenges-workbook

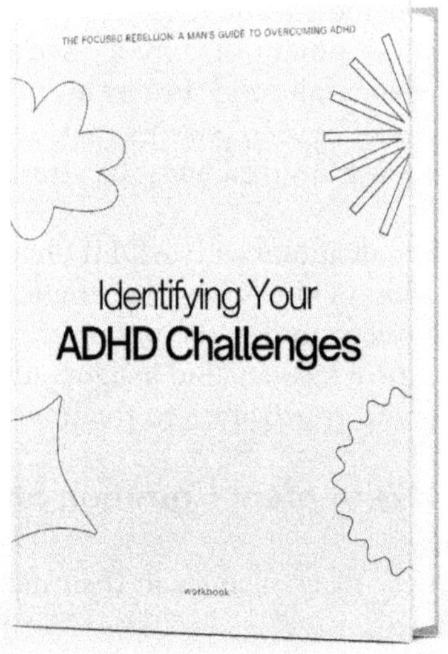

The Strengths of ADHD in Men: Harnessing the Positive Aspects of ADHD

While ADHD can present various challenges for men, it is essential to recognize that there are also positive aspects and potential strengths associated with the disorder. By embracing these unique traits, men with ADHD can harness their potential and thrive in various aspects of their lives. Here are some positive aspects and potential strengths of ADHD in men:

Creativity and divergent thinking: Men with ADHD often exhibit exceptional creativity and divergent thinking abilities. They can generate original ideas, think outside the box, and approach problems from unique perspectives. These qualities can be valuable in artistic pursuits, entrepreneurship, and innovative problem-solving situations.

High energy levels: Hyperactivity, often seen as a challenge, can also be a strength when channeled effectively. Men with ADHD can possess high energy levels, enabling them to be productive and engaged in activities they are passionate about. This trait can be particularly beneficial in fast-paced or physically demanding careers.

Resilience: Living with ADHD and overcoming its challenges can foster resilience in men with the disorder. They may develop a stronger ability to bounce back from setbacks and adapt to change, which can be advantageous in both personal and professional situations.

Empathy and emotional sensitivity: Some men with ADHD may possess heightened emotional sensitivity, allowing them to empathize with others and form deep connections. This trait can be valuable in careers that require strong interpersonal skills, such as counseling, social work, or healthcare.

Unique problem-solving abilities: Due to their divergent thinking and atypical cognitive processing, men with ADHD may excel at finding unique solutions to problems or identifying opportunities that others may overlook. This ability can make them valuable contributors in various professional settings.

Finding the Funny Side: Leveraging Humor for Men with ADHD
Maintaining a sense of humor can be beneficial for men with ADHD, as it can help reduce stress, build resilience, and foster a positive outlook on life. Here are some ways to inject humor into daily life:

Laugh at yourself: Embrace your quirks and learn to laugh at the occasional missteps that come with ADHD. This self-deprecating humor can help you maintain perspective and keep your challenges in check.

Surround yourself with humor: Engage with humorous content, such as comedy shows, funny movies, or stand-up comedians. These can provide a much-needed distraction from daily stressors and help you cultivate a more lighthearted approach to life.

Share your experiences: Connect with others who have ADHD and share your humorous stories and experiences. This camaraderie can help you feel less alone and allow you to find humor in the shared challenges of living with ADHD.

Practice finding the humor in everyday situations: Train yourself to identify the humor in everyday life. This can help you develop a more positive outlook and enhance your ability to cope with the challenges of ADHD.

ADHD in men presents unique challenges and experiences shaped by factors such as biological differences, societal expectations, and individual life circumstances. By understanding these differences, healthcare professionals, educators, and support networks can develop tailored strategies and interventions to address the specific needs of men with ADHD.

Furthermore, recognizing and embracing the positive aspects and potential strengths associated with ADHD can help men build self-acceptance, foster resilience, and thrive in their personal and professional lives. By maintaining a sense of humor and focusing on their unique abilities, men with ADHD can cultivate a more balanced perspective on their disorder, empowering them to overcome challenges and embrace their potential.

Mindfulness for Men with ADHD: Cultivating Self-Awareness and Compassion

Mindfulness is the practice of intentionally focusing on the present moment with a non-judgmental attitude, which can be especially advantageous for men with ADHD. Implementing mindfulness techniques can support men with ADHD in various ways:

Cultivating self-awareness: Mindfulness enables men to develop a deeper understanding of their thoughts, emotions, and behaviors. This enhanced self-awareness allows them to identify ADHD-related patterns and create targeted strategies to address these challenges.

Curbing impulsivity: By promoting increased self-awareness, mindfulness empowers men with ADHD to pause and reflect before reacting, resulting in reduced impulsive behaviors and more thoughtful decision-making.

Managing emotions: Incorporating mindfulness practices, such as meditation or deep breathing exercises, can equip men with ADHD with the tools to better regulate their emotions and mitigate emotional volatility.

Sharpening focus: Employing mindfulness techniques can help men with ADHD hone their concentration and attention skills, leading to heightened productivity and successful task completion.

Fostering compassion: Mindfulness encourages men with ADHD to adopt a more compassionate and non-judgmental outlook towards themselves and their ADHD symptoms, nurturing self-acceptance and boosting self-esteem.

By integrating mindfulness practices into their daily routines, men with ADHD can effectively manage their symptoms and enhance their overall well-being.

CHAPTER 5: FOSTERING FOCUS: ENHANCING TIME MANAGEMENT AND CONCENTRATION SKILLS

The Importance of Time Management and Concentration Skills for Men with ADHD

For men with ADHD, mastering time management and concentration skills can be life-changing. ADHD often leads to procrastination, disorganization, and difficulty staying on task, which can impact various aspects of daily life, from work to personal relationships. Developing strategies to improve these skills can significantly enhance productivity, self-esteem, and overall quality of life.

Time Management Techniques for Men with ADHD

a. The Pomodoro Technique: The Pomodoro Technique involves breaking work into short, focused intervals (called "Pomodoros") with short breaks in between. This method can help men with ADHD stay on task without feeling overwhelmed. To implement this technique, choose a task, set a timer for 25 minutes, work on the task until the timer rings, take a 5-minute break, and repeat. After four Pomodoros, take a longer break (15-30 minutes).

WHAT IS THE POMODORO TECHNIQUE?

A method for staying focused and mentally fresh

STEP 1 — Pick a task

STEP 2 — Set a 25-minute timer

STEP 3 — Work on your task until the time is up

STEP 4 — Take a 5-minute break

STEP 5 — Every 4 pomodoros, take a longer 15-30 minute break

b. Time Blocking: Time blocking is the practice of dedicating specific time slots to particular tasks or activities. This strategy can help men with ADHD create structure and manage their time more efficiently. Start by assessing your daily and weekly priorities, and then schedule time blocks for each task in your calendar. Remember to include buffer time for unexpected events or distractions.

c. Prioritization and Task Lists: Creating a prioritized task list can help men with ADHD focus on their most important tasks and avoid getting overwhelmed. Begin by listing all your tasks and responsibilities, then prioritize them based on importance and urgency. Use the Eisenhower Matrix to categorize tasks into four quadrants: urgent and important, important but not urgent, urgent but not important, and neither urgent nor important. Focus on completing tasks in the first two quadrants first.

Improving Concentration and Reducing Distractions

a. Creating an ADHD-Friendly Environment: Designing a workspace that minimizes distractions can improve focus for men with ADHD. Consider using noise-canceling headphones, decluttering your workspace, and removing any unnecessary items that may be visually distracting. Experiment with different environments to find what works best for you.

b. Mindfulness Techniques for Improved Focus: Mindfulness practices, such as meditation, can help men with ADHD increase their concentration and self-awareness. Try a simple mindfulness exercise: Sit comfortably, close your eyes, and focus on your breath for 5-10 minutes. When your mind wanders, gently bring your attention back to your breath. Practice this exercise daily to improve your ability to focus.

c. The Role of Exercise and Nutrition in Enhancing Concentration: Regular exercise and a balanced diet can help improve concentration for men with ADHD. Physical activity increases blood flow to the brain, potentially improving cognitive function. Additionally, consuming a diet rich in whole foods, lean proteins, and healthy fats can support brain health and improve focus.

Practical Time Management and Concentration Exercises

a. Time Management Exercise: The Weekly Planning Session: Set aside 30 minutes each week to plan your upcoming tasks and activities. Use your prioritized task list, time blocks, and calendar to create a detailed schedule. Review your plan daily and adjust as needed.

b. Concentration Exercise: The Focus-Boosting Meditation: Practice a 10-minute guided meditation designed to improve focus and concentration. Apps like Headspace and Calm offer a variety of focus-oriented meditations. Consistent practice can lead to long-term improvements in concentration.

Recommended Resources and Tools for Time Management and Concentration

a. Books:

- "Getting Things Done" by David Allen
- "The One Thing" by Gary Keller and Jay Papasan
- "Deep Work" by Cal Newport

b. Websites:

- RescueTime (time management app): www.rescuetime.com
- Toggl Track (time tracking app): www.toggl.com
- Todoist (task management app): www.todoist.com

c. Apps:

- Focus@Will (music designed to improve focus): www.focusatwill.com
- Forest (app to reduce phone distractions): www.forestapp.cc
- Brain.fm (AI-generated music to enhance focus): www.brain.fm

These resources, techniques, and exercises can help men with ADHD improve their time management and concentration skills, leading to a more fulfilling and productive life.

Remember, practice and consistency are key to mastering these skills.

CHAPTER 6: EXPLORING TREATMENT OPTIONS: MEDICATION, THERAPY, AND LIFESTYLE CHANGES

Understanding the different types of medications for ADHD
ADHD medications can be a game-changer for many men struggling with the condition. They generally fall into two categories: stimulants and non-stimulants.

a. Stimulants: These medications work by increasing the levels of certain neurotransmitters in the brain, improving focus and reducing impulsivity. Some common stimulant medications include:

- Methylphenidate (Ritalin, Concerta)
- Amphetamine (Adderall, Vyvanse)

b. Non-Stimulants: These medications can be a good alternative for those who cannot tolerate stimulants or have certain medical conditions. Some common non-stimulant medications include:

- Atomoxetine (Strattera)
- Guanfacine (Intuniv)
- Clonidine (Kapvay)

Pros and cons of medication for ADHD treatment

Pros:
- Can provide significant improvements in focus, organization, and impulse control
- Fast-acting, with effects usually noticeable within hours or days of starting treatment

Cons:
- Potential side effects, such as sleep disturbances, appetite changes, and increased heart rate
- Not a cure-all; may need to be combined with therapy or lifestyle changes for optimal results

ADHD therapy options: Cognitive Behavioral Therapy (CBT), psychotherapy, and coaching

a. Cognitive Behavioral Therapy (CBT): CBT is a short-term, goal-oriented therapy that focuses on changing negative thought patterns and behaviors. It can help men with ADHD develop coping strategies, improve time management, and reduce symptoms.

b. Psychotherapy: This form of talk therapy can help men with ADHD explore the emotional impact of their condition, improve self-esteem, and build better relationships.

c. Coaching: ADHD coaching is a supportive, non-judgmental process that focuses on helping individuals set goals, develop strategies, and stay accountable. Coaches can provide practical guidance on managing ADHD symptoms in daily life.

CHAPTER 7: CRAFTING YOUR PERSONALIZED PLAN: TAILORING ADHD MANAGEMENT STRATEGIES

1. Assessing your unique ADHD symptoms and challenges

Before you can craft your personalized ADHD management plan, it's essential to take stock of your specific symptoms and challenges. Write down the aspects of ADHD that impact your life the most, such as disorganization, impulsivity, or difficulty concentrating. This self-assessment will serve as a foundation for building a tailored plan that addresses your unique needs.

2. Identifying your strengths and leveraging them in your ADHD management plan

ADHD isn't all doom and gloom! Many men with ADHD have unique strengths, such as creativity, enthusiasm, and resilience. Identify your strengths and consider how they can be used to your advantage in managing ADHD. For example, if you're a natural problem-solver, leverage that skill to find innovative solutions to your ADHD challenges.

3. Setting realistic goals and priorities for your ADHD treatment

Now that you know your symptoms and strengths, set realistic and achievable goals for your ADHD management. Focus on what matters most to you and prioritize the areas that need the most improvement. Break larger goals into smaller, manageable steps and celebrate your progress along the way.

4. Combining medication, therapy, and lifestyle changes for a holistic approach

A well-rounded ADHD management plan often includes a combination of medication, therapy, and lifestyle changes. Consult with your healthcare team to determine the best treatment options for your specific needs. Incorporate daily exercise, healthy eating habits, and stress reduction techniques to support your overall well-being.

5. Developing a daily routine to support your ADHD management

Establishing a consistent daily routine can be incredibly beneficial for men with ADHD. This routine should include designated times for work, leisure, exercise, and sleep. Stick to your routine as much as possible, but don't be too hard on yourself if things don't always go as planned.

6. Building a support network: Friends, family, and professionals

Having a solid support network is crucial for long-term ADHD management. Communicate openly with friends and family members about your ADHD and enlist their help when needed. Stay connected with your healthcare team and consider joining a support group or working with an ADHD coach for additional guidance.

7. Adjusting your plan as needed: Tracking progress and making changes

Your ADHD management plan should be flexible and adaptable to your changing needs. Regularly assess your progress and make adjustments as necessary. If a particular strategy isn't working, don't be afraid to try something new.

8. Embracing self-compassion and patience throughout your ADHD journey

Managing ADHD is a lifelong process, and it's essential to practice patience and self-compassion along the way. Remember that setbacks are a normal part of the journey, and you're not alone in your struggles. Keep a sense of humor, stay committed to your goals, and celebrate your successes, no matter how small they may seem.

CHAPTER 8: SUCCESS STORIES: INSPIRING TALES OF MEN THRIVING WITH ADHD

Every hero needs an inspiring tale. Success stories of men thriving with ADHD can motivate and encourage others to face their own challenges head-on. These real-life examples show how individuals have harnessed their ADHD traits and overcome obstacles to achieve great things. As you read these stories, remember that you too can write your own success story.

The Entrepreneurial Spirit

Meet Dave, a successful entrepreneur with ADHD. Dave has always been full of ideas, and he quickly realized that his creative and high-energy nature was perfect for starting his own business. Instead of seeing his ADHD as a roadblock, Dave embraced it as an advantage in the fast-paced world of entrepreneurship. His ability to think outside the box and take calculated risks has helped him build a thriving business empire. The key takeaway from Dave's story? Don't let ADHD hold you back—use it to fuel your dreams!

Athletic Achievement

James, an accomplished athlete, didn't let ADHD get in the way of his passion for sports. Despite facing challenges with focus and impulsivity, he discovered that intense physical activity helped him manage his symptoms. James dedicated himself to rigorous training and harnessed his competitive nature to excel in his chosen sport. Today, he's a role model for others with ADHD, proving that with determination and hard work, anything is possible.

The Art of ADHD

For some, ADHD is a catalyst for creativity. Take Alex, an artist who credits his ADHD for his unique artistic style and boundless imagination. Instead of being limited by his challenges, Alex turned them into a source of inspiration, using his intense emotions and energy to fuel his creative expression. By embracing his ADHD traits, he gained recognition in the art world and inspired others to see the beauty in their own differences.

Education and Empathy

Tom, a dedicated educator, understands ADHD from both personal and professional perspectives. He uses his firsthand experiences to help students with ADHD succeed in the classroom. By implementing teaching strategies tailored to their needs, Tom has made a significant impact on his students' educational outcomes. His story shows that understanding and empathy can go a long way in helping others overcome challenges.

Building Strong Relationships

Life with ADHD can be challenging, but as Mike's story demonstrates, it doesn't have to be a barrier to strong relationships and family life. Mike learned to communicate openly about his ADHD with his partner, and together they developed strategies to manage his symptoms. His resilience and commitment to personal growth have made him a loving partner and father, proving that ADHD doesn't define your capacity for love and connection.

Learning from Others

The stories shared here offer valuable lessons on perseverance, resilience, and self-acceptance. Each individual found unique ways to harness their ADHD traits and turn them into strengths. Remember that these success stories are not just about the achievements themselves, but the journey it took to reach them.

Your Own ADHD Journey

As you reflect on the stories shared in this chapter, consider how they might apply to your own life. What can you learn from these individuals' experiences? How can you use their strategies to overcome your own challenges and embrace your ADHD traits? Remember, your story is still being written, and you have the power to make it a success story of your own.

CHAPTER 9: ESSENTIAL RESOURCES: BOOKS, WEBSITES, APPS, AND SUPPORT GROUPS FOR MEN WITH ADHD

Recommended Books

A well-rounded reading list can be an invaluable resource for men with ADHD. These books can provide insights, strategies, and inspiration to help you better understand and manage your ADHD. Some popular titles include:

- "Delivered from Distraction" by Edward M. Hallowell and John J. Ratey
- "ADD-Friendly Ways to Organize Your Life" by Judith Kolberg and Kathleen Nadeau
- "The ADHD Advantage" by Dale Archer
- "Mastering Your Adult ADHD" by Steven A. Safren, Susan E. Sprich, and Carol A. Perlman
- "More Attention, Less Deficit" by Ari Tuckman

Useful Websites and Online Resources

There are many websites and online resources available to help men with ADHD access valuable information, tools, and support. Some of the top websites include:

- ADDitude Magazine (www.additudemag.com)
- CHADD (Children and Adults with Attention-Deficit/Hyperactivity Disorder) (www.chadd.org)
- ADHD & You (www.adhdandyou.com)
- TotallyADD (www.totallyadd.com)
- HelpGuide (www.helpguide.org)

Apps for Managing ADHD

Modern technology offers a wide variety of apps designed to help those with ADHD manage their symptoms and daily tasks. Some popular apps include:

- Todoist (Task management)
- Evernote (Note-taking and organization)
- Focus@Will (Focus-enhancing music)
- RescueTime (Time management and productivity tracking)
- Headspace (Meditation and mindfulness)

Support Groups and Forums

Connecting with others who share similar experiences and challenges can be incredibly beneficial for men with ADHD. Support groups and forums can provide a safe space to share stories, advice, and encouragement. Some notable options include:

- ADDA (Attention Deficit Disorder Association) (www.add.org)
- National Resource Center on ADHD (www.help4adhd.org)
- ADHD Reddit community (www.reddit.com/r/ADHD)
- The ADHD Support Group on Facebook
- Meetup.com (Search for local ADHD support groups in your area)

Working with Professionals

Don't hesitate to seek help from professionals such as therapists, psychiatrists, or ADHD coaches. These experts can provide guidance, support, and resources tailored to your specific needs. Reach out to local mental health clinics or search online directories to find professionals specializing in ADHD.

By exploring and utilizing these resources, you can expand your ADHD management toolkit and connect with a supportive community.

CHAPTER 10: STAYING MOTIVATED: COMMITTING TO LONG-TERM ADHD MANAGEMENT AND GOAL PURSUIT.

Managing ADHD is a journey that requires patience, perseverance, and consistent effort. In this chapter, we'll explore essential strategies for staying motivated, committed, and resilient in your pursuit of personal and professional goals. By utilizing the workbook exercises provided, you can customize these strategies to your unique needs and circumstances and track your progress along the way.

Setting Realistic Goals

Goal setting is a critical component of managing ADHD. It provides direction, focus, and motivation. However, setting unrealistic goals can lead to frustration, disappointment, and burnout. It's important to set achievable and realistic goals, break them down into smaller, manageable tasks, and adjust expectations when necessary. In the workbook exercises, you'll learn how to set SMART goals and create an action plan to achieve them.

Tracking Progress

Tracking progress is essential for staying motivated and celebrating small wins. It's a tangible way to measure your progress, hold yourself accountable, and recognize your accomplishments. There are various methods for tracking progress, such as journaling, using apps, or creating visual representations of accomplishments. In the workbook exercises, you'll find templates and prompts to help you track your progress and celebrate your successes.

Building a Support System

Building a support system is critical for managing ADHD successfully. It's essential to have friends, family, professionals, and peers who understand and support your ADHD journey. Your support system can provide encouragement, accountability, and practical assistance. In the workbook exercises, you'll learn how to cultivate and maintain these relationships and communicate your needs effectively.

Embracing Flexibility

Flexibility is key to staying resilient and motivated in the face of setbacks and challenges. It's essential to adapt to changes and adjust your strategies as needed. The workbook exercises will guide you in developing a flexible mindset and staying motivated despite obstacles.

Self-Compassion and Mindfulness

Self-compassion and mindfulness are powerful tools for managing ADHD long-term. Practicing self-compassion and mindfulness can help reduce stress, enhance self-awareness, and promote emotional regulation. In the workbook exercises, you'll learn techniques for cultivating self-compassion and mindfulness, such as self-reflective prompts and mindfulness meditations.

Maintaining Healthy Habits

Maintaining healthy habits is essential for sustainable ADHD management. Regular exercise, a balanced diet, and sufficient sleep can help enhance focus, energy, and overall well-being. In the workbook exercises, you'll learn how to create and maintain healthy habits and develop a self-care plan.

Continuous Learning and Growth

Continuous learning and growth are critical for managing ADHD throughout life. Staying informed about new research, treatment options, and strategies for managing ADHD can help you stay on top of your condition and enhance your quality of life. In the workbook exercises, you'll find resources and prompts for continuous learning and growth.

By utilizing the workbook exercises provided, you can customize these strategies to your unique needs and circumstances and track your progress along the way. With commitment, perseverance, and self-awareness, you can stay motivated, manage your ADHD, and achieve your personal and professional goals.

CHAPTER 11: THE JOURNEY AHEAD: REFLECTIONS AND ENCOURAGEMENT FOR MEN WITH ADHD

As we come to the end of this guide, I want to acknowledge the hard work and dedication that has brought you to this point. Managing ADHD is no easy feat, and it takes time, patience, and commitment to make progress. Whether you're just starting your journey or have been managing ADHD for years, I hope this guide has provided you with valuable insights, strategies, and encouragement.

Remember that you are not alone in your struggles. Millions of men around the world face similar challenges and are working hard to manage their ADHD. It's important to reach out for help when you need it and to build a support network of friends, family, and professionals who can offer guidance and support.

As you move forward on your ADHD journey, keep in mind that progress is not always linear. There will be ups and downs, setbacks and successes. It's important to embrace self-compassion and patience along the way, and to celebrate the small victories along with the big ones.

Above all, I want to encourage you not to give up. With the right tools, strategies, and mindset, it's possible to manage ADHD and live a fulfilling and meaningful life. So take what you've learned in this guide, use it to craft your personalized ADHD management plan, and move forward with confidence, resilience, and determination.

Thank you for allowing me to be a part of your journey, and I wish you all the best as you continue to overcome the challenges of ADHD and live your best life.

REFERENCES

American Psychiatric Association. (2013). Diagnostic and Statistical Manual of Mental Disorders (5th ed.). Arlington, VA: American Psychiatric Publishing.

Quinn, P. O., & Madhoo, M. (2014). A review of attention-deficit/hyperactivity disorder in women and girls: uncovering this hidden diagnosis. The primary care companion for CNS disorders, 16(3).

Willcutt, E. G. (2012). The prevalence of DSM-IV attention-deficit/hyperactivity disorder: a meta-analytic review. Neurotherapeutics, 9(3), 490-499.

Rucklidge, J. J. (2010). Gender differences in attention-deficit/hyperactivity disorder. Psychiatric Clinics, 33(2), 357-373.

Gudjonsson, G. H., Sigurdsson, J. F., Adalsteinsson, T. F., & Young, S. (2013). The relationship between ADHD symptoms, mood instability, and self-reported offending. Journal of Attention Disorders, 17(4), 339-346.

Kessler, R. C., Adler, L., Barkley, R., Biederman, J., Conners, C. K., Demler, O., ... & Spencer, T. (2006). The prevalence and correlates of adult ADHD in the United States: results from the National Comorbidity Survey Replication. American Journal of Psychiatry, 163(4), 716-723.

Stevens, K., Surís, A., Clavenna, A., & Khanna, R. (2016). The role of childhood emotional abuse in the development of adult ADHD symptoms: A comparison of three racial/ethnic groups. Journal of Attention Disorders, 20(2), 107-117.

Teicher, M. H., Samson, J. A., Polcari, A., & McGreenery, C. E. (2016). Sticks, stones, and hurtful words: Relative effects of various forms of childhood maltreatment. American Journal of Psychiatry, 173(9), 907-913.

White, H. A., & Shah, P. (2011). Creative style and achievement in adults with attention-deficit/hyperactivity disorder. Personality and Individual Differences, 50(5), 673-677.

Nadeau, K. G., & Quinn, P. O. (Eds.). (2019). ADHD in Adults: What the Science Says. Guilford Publications.

Wymbs, B. T., Pelham, W. E., Molina, B. S. G., & Gnagy, E. M. (2008). Mother and adolescent reports of interparental discord among families of adolescents with and without attention-deficit/hyperactivity disorder. Journal of Emotional and Behavioral Disorders, 16(1), 29-41.

Englar-Carlson, M., & Kiselica, M. S. (2013). Affirming the strengths in men: A positive masculinity approach to assisting male clients. Journal of Counseling & Development, 91(4), 399-409.

Barkley, R. A. (2015). Attention deficit hyperactivity disorder: a handbook for diagnosis and treatment (4th ed.). Guilford Press.

Keller, G., & Papasan, J. (2012). The One Thing: The Surprisingly Simple Truth Behind Extraordinary Results. Bard Press.

Newport, C. (2016). Deep Work: Rules for Focused Success